Elder Reflections
for People Who Care

by Pat Nekola

First Edition

ISBN: 0-9660610-6-3

Library of Congress Cataloging Number: 2003108328

Cover by: Carol Calabro

Published by:
Applewood Ink
A division of: Catering by Design
P.O. Box 181
Waukesha, WI 53187

Dedication

I would like to dedicate this book to all the beautiful, elderly people who have shared their stories, reflections, and memories that carried them through their life. They have left their "touch" on my life forever.

I would also like to remember my Grandma Evans (my father's mother). She was a rock in my life. She took time from her busy schedule to teach me many life-skill lessons, which have helped my faith to grow. I have carried these lessons with me through my entire life.

Acknowledgments

I want to thank my husband, Steve, for his continued patience and support (both spiritual and financial) during my writing. Thank you for loving me.

To my extended family and birthday group, the Lesch, Kramer, and Bell families, thank you for always caring.

Thanks, also, to *Graphic Liaisons, LLC*, for their dedication and understanding in preparing my manuscripts for publication.

Introduction

As Pat Nekola traveled the country working with the elderly, she became inspired to write down the stories they told her and the occasions they shared together. As she listened to them she gained much wisdom and insight into life.

Pat has included stories about her grandmother, Barbara Evans, and also about her mother, who suffered with Alzheimer's Disease. She has stories from working in care facilities and also from the staff at her parish. Pat has helped train Girl Scouts and other young adults to do intergenerational programs and use their creative abilities to get involved in activities with Alzheimer's patients to help them stay as vital as possible.

This book is designed for families and caregivers. Don't forget to take time for respite care for yourself. You are doing a most difficult job of caring for an elder parent or someone in a nursing facility. Pat hopes this book will inspire you and carry you through those difficult times as a caregiver.

Contents

"It is in giving that you shall receive.
Remember that love is the greatest gift of all.
Give your love and you will
receive the love in return."

—Author unknown

Grandma Evans

Grandma Evans ran a noodle business in the late '50s and early '60s, even though she was blind. She was an amazing woman! She called it "Ma Evans Homemade Noodles". The noodles were made from scratch. She mixed up big batches of dough and rolled them out to perfection. After the noodles were dry she rolled them up in a diploma-like fashion and cut each noodle to the same thickness. She had a very sharp knife to accomplish this task. Even being blind, she never cut herself. She had special bags and labels that said, "Ma Evans Homemade Noodles". Our family helped weigh out the noodles into one-pound packages, and I had the responsibility of assisting her in putting labels on the bags and sealing them. My uncle would deliver the noodles to the local grocery stores. Grandma charged fifty cents more a bag for her noodles than for "store-bought" noodles but she never had any trouble selling her noodles.

When we would take a break we shared an orange. I treasure these times, for Grandma was teaching me some good sound values—without me even realizing this was a lesson.

She told me that God's assignment to parents was to raise their family to the best of their ability. It was a parent's responsibility to teach each child real-life skills to help them to become good sound citizens. She said, "Pat, you need to give your children wings to fly away on their own. Please understand those wings will fly back to see you, and will willingly care for you if you have carried through with your job as a good strong parent." She

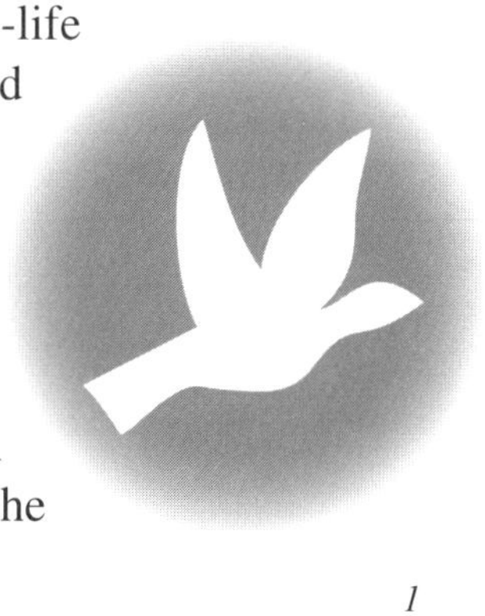

was right, too, because her children came often to visit and helped her until her death.

She also taught me to reach out to the needy and to be kind to people. She said, "It is in giving that you receive. Remember, what goes around—comes around."

I thank my grandmother daily for being a big influence in my life.

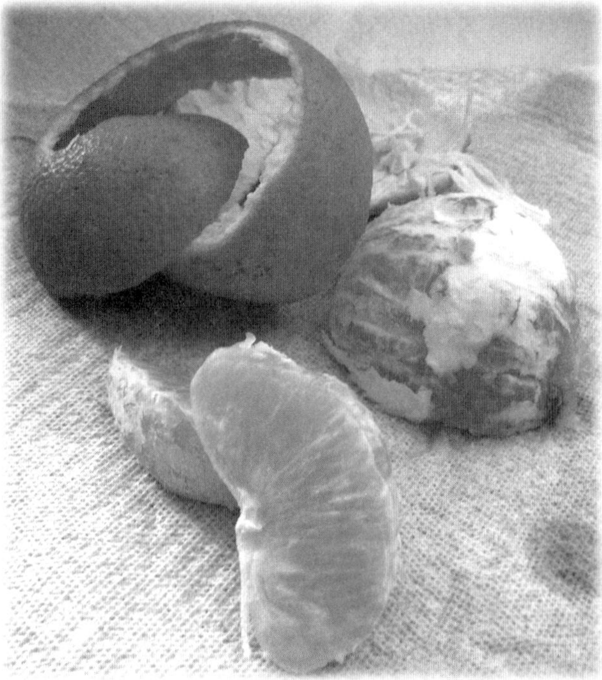

Country Music

I visited a gentleman on a one-on-one visit in his room in a care facility. He had the radio tuned in to country music. I asked him why he listened to country music and his reply was that country music artists speak of family, religion, our country, patriotism, and pride. He had served in World War II and was very patriotic.

When I did my next program I asked the residents how many liked country music. Several hands went up so I asked if they would share some of their favorite country songs and artists with the group.

That afternoon I went shopping for country music. Shortly after that I planned a western picnic and played country western songs for the residents. They thoroughly enjoyed the event.

Two songs the elderly enjoy are, "Hey, Good Lookin'" and "King of the Road".

Note: I thought if I keep entertaining in care facilities soon the baby boomers will be taking the place of the current residents. I'll have to get with it again and learn their music for their enjoyment. THAT WILL BE SOMETHING ALL RIGHT!

Millie's Story

A business had donated one dozen computers to a care facility and Millie was invited to take part in a computer class. Of course, she was reluctant at first. But after some coaxing she joined the class. Each person had an assignment, and Millie was surprised how much she was learning. It was fun and she felt part of a team.

One day she was rushed to the hospital and was confined to bed until she regained her health. Her heart ached because she was missing her computer class. She felt she was letting her classmates down and she needed to get her assignment completed. All day she thought about how she could get back to the care facility and complete her computer work. After a time the nurse came to see Millie and asked her, "Millie, what are you doing out of bed?"

"You don't understand," Millie replied, "I am taking a computer class and I need to get my assignment finished." Millie begged the nurse to help her complete her assignment. When the work was complete the nurse helped Millie back to bed, and delivered the work to the care facility on her way home.

Two days later Millie was well enough to return to the care facility. When the other residents saw Millie they gave her a standing round of applause! She was so proud—and happy to be one of the group of computer students.

Answered Prayer

One day I visited a minister who was recovering from a stroke. He was doing very well. I asked him about his feelings on God and prayer.

His answer was, "Please remember that God always answers your prayers. He may not answer them the way you think He should, but instead He answers them in your best interest."

It made me think about how God had called me to the mission of helping Alzheimer's patients, due to my own mother becoming afflicted with the disease. I reflected for a moment and said a prayer of thanks.

Al

Al has Alzheimer's Disease.

I've found the elderly like to hear about the weather, and it is usually a good topic to break the ice.

One day I proceeded to say that it was a really hot day, and how many of the residents remembered "Dog Days" in summer?

Al usually came to our activities, but he rarely said anything—he was outnumbered by the ladies. (This is true in most care facilities.) But on this day as I was talking about "Dog Days" he spontaneously called out, "Boy! It is so hot. I sure could go for an ice-cold beer right now!"

I knew something had triggered his memory—he was thinking.

Victoria's Story

Victoria was born in Buchloe, Germany, in 1910. She was orphaned at a very young age. At the age of 20 she found a sponsor and came to the United States, where she met the man that became her husband. He always kidded her that he had to come to America to meet a beautiful German lady.

Victoria had a big heart and was always helping people. She loved to bake—at Easter she would make lamb cakes and give them away for gifts. At Christmas she made German cookies and many sweet breads and she would take the treats with her to work. She also made greeting cards and loved flowers.

I met Victoria while working at a care facility. She was afflicted with a stroke and had aphasia. She could not speak, but she understood every word that was said to her. Her family members were very strong advocates for Victoria. Her daughter brought her to one of the Halloween parties at the facility. I took a picture of the two of them together as a memory. Every Wednesday morning her son would visit. Victoria always had a smile about her and a gentleness that a person could not miss.

I would hold her hand as I walked with her. Sometimes we went out to lunch with several other residents. She loved the German music and played the simple version of Bingo.

Here's a poem about Victoria that I wrote after her death.

Sweet Lovely Victoria

You won my heart
Right from the start.

You showed every person you cared,
Especially your loved ones,
With whom your talents you shared.

Nothing was too much for you to bear.
When asked for your help
You were willing to give,
To help greatly for mankind to live.

A radiant smile
Was simply your style,
As you went that extra mile.

So rest, sweet Victoria, rest,
Knowing on earth
You did your best.

Until we meet again in heaven,
As I walk around the pearl-strewn bend
To greet you, please know Victoria
You have touched my heart.

Helen's Story

I knew Helen back in the old days when I catered parties for the Womens' Club. She was community minded. As she grew older she wasn't taking proper care of herself. She lived alone and wasn't eating right. Her family insisted she should be placed at a care facility, and she reluctantly moved. While her physical health improved she suffered from some depression. She felt isolated from the community she so loved. She was still very mentally alert and had been a busy person all her life. Now, she was sitting idle with everything being done for her.

One day I went to her room and told her I needed help. I had bulletin boards in the facility that needed to be changed and updated each month. I also had cards that needed to be sorted and hymn books to be assembled. I told her I could not keep up with all the work.

"That is when I thought of you, Helen," I continued. "I would be so appreciative if you could just help a little bit." I promised her I would do things for her in return as a trade if she could help me out.

She agreed to help me, and her first assignment was sorting the greeting cards that been donated to the facility. She sorted them according to season, and then she got the idea to sell the cards for twenty-five cents each. This change would purchase juice or soda for people attending our activity programs.

Then she assembled the hymn books and also some of the one-on-one books used by the Alzheimer's patients. She kept the bulletin boards updated until she became terminally ill. She even got the entire staff to bring in pictures for the bulletin boards.

One day her daughter from Texas called to talk to Helen, but she politely told her daughter to call back as she was too busy working to talk then. She was working on an urgent job at the time—she was working for me! (It wasn't until after her death that I learned of this incident.)

Helen's entire family thanked me for helping their mom stay busy and feel needed. By helping me and feeling important—she was no longer depressed. Everyone needs to be needed throughout their entire life.

Over the Hill?

Mike's dad, John, was living in a care facility, and Mike visited often. This day John was a little grumpy and he complained of getting old.

On his next visit Mike brought John a T-shirt with this message:

You are now over the hill.
Where?
What?
When?
I never saw the hill!

He got a smile from his dad. John had been a good sport all of his life and could take some kidding good naturedly.

Nancy's Story

Nancy was dying of cancer and was in terrible pain. The doctor had ordered the staff to keep her comfortable. As I made my rounds each day, I always visited Nancy. I said prayers with her and listened to her wisdom.

"Honey," she would say, "I know I'll be on this earth until God calls me home. I want to go home now, but I must wait on His time. I am ready to go to heaven. My family has been wonderful to me. We have always been close and have enjoyed visiting and playing games."

Nancy was only seven when her mother died of cancer, and she prayed daily that she would live long enough to see her daughters grown. God granted her wish.

Nancy continued, "My husband was a good family man and took good care of us. Please, pray for me that God will call me home soon."

Nancy was a gentle lady. She taught me a lot about patience.

A prayer from an elder person—

Dear Lord,

These weary bones cannot continue to carry me. I have run many miles and had much happiness throughout my life. While I no longer can see, I can envision seeing and sitting with you, dear God.

Please, Lord, speak to me and call me home. I am ready to be with you.

—Amen

Katie's Story

Katie lived to be 100 years old. I visited her often. Even at 100 she was beautiful. She had a great attitude about life. She kept her memory until the last three years of her life. Her past was very interesting to me.

At age 23 Katie became a beauty queen. She spoke of the thrill of winning, but how she felt so responsible to represent her state. The gentleman that was her escort for the beauty pageant was a "lady's man". She fell for him and they were married. The marriage ended in divorce, so she attended school and learned to be a secretary.

She would always say, "When things go to sour grapes, turn them into sweet-smelling wine and taste the goodness. Now go forward and don't look back."

She loved music, dancing, and good times. She always thanked me for coming and visiting her and playing my accordion. She loved the song "K, K, K, Katy" and requested it every week.

We had a big cake and celebrated for her 100th birthday. She dressed up and had a beautiful corsage. She really enjoyed her big day. One month after her party, she died in her sleep.

The music brought Katie to life. Music is truly God's gift to help the inner soul of mankind. It was so wonderful to watch Katie sing and motion with her hands in time with the music.

The Teddy Bear Story

While working as an Activity Director I met another Director who was very talented. She put her activity ideas together in book form.

She showed me how to make teddy bears. (About two years later I modified the pattern and started making bears. I used flannel, cotton, and other soft fabrics.)

As I began to work with the Alzheimer's patients I realized that bears were a big hit. I approached my pastor and requested a spot in the church bulletin to ask others to bring fabrics, stuffing, and ribbons for the bears. The parish members responded with zest. I even got some volunteers to help cut out the fabric and sew the bears.

Our local Adult Day Care Center clients stuffed and hand sewed the back opening closed on the bears, and they were delivered to many care facilities as an on-going project. Bears were also shipped to the Alzheimer's Association in South Carolina and Ohio. When I visited other facilities to present programs the bears always went with me, when we passed them out to the residents it was so exciting to witness their reactions.

At one facility I was informed that Robert never spoke—not a word, let alone a sentence! He was a very short man with a slight build. As I passed out the bears I asked him to pick one for himself, and he did. Then he got up from his assigned seat and preceded to show off his bear saying, "Look at my bear!" repeatedly. The staff was shocked to see him speaking, and it was so touching I could hardly hold back my tears.

At another facility I walked room-to-room doing one-on-one visits and handing out bears. I gave a bear to Erma, and she smiled—ever so slightly. She hugged and kissed the bear, "Oh Willie, Willie, Willie!" she exclaimed.

I asked, "Who is Willie?"

"Willie is my baby."

"Where is Willie?"

"Willie is in heaven. He is my angel."

Later I learned that Erma had lost her son, Willie, at birth. Even though she had Alzheimer's the pain was still there.

I learned that even with memory loss there are some things patients still remember and we need to deal with this situation as it arises. This is where reminiscence (an indulgence in painful memories) can help bring closure to this tragedy.

Erma was still grieving, after all those years had passed. (I asked her questions about Willie to try to walk her through the grieving process—Who, What, How, When.)

The bear program has been so successful we continue to make and distribute them. My neighbor is a very talented seamstress. She has sewn the majority of the bears, and the clients at Adult Day Care really enjoy helping. This is a team effort that can bring joy to Alzheimer's patients.

May's Story

It seems that when May was born her father didn't want her because she wasn't a boy. He did not treat her very well. Two years later she had a brother. Everything went for the son of the family and there was nothing for May.

At age 7, May's parents were killed and her aunt took her brother to raise, but declined to take May.

At last her mother's friend provided a good home for May and May stayed with her until she finished high school.

May married at an early age to a wonderful man and they raised twins. She would say, "God will never give you more than you can handle, and He will provide only if you have faith."

A Recipe for Life

by Pat Nekola

Heaping cups of love.
1 bundle of faith, hope, and charity.
Several pinches of kindness.
1 gallon of thoughtfulness.
1 peck of strength.
1 pound of enthusiasm.
Bouquet Garni of moral character, hard labor, and patience.

Practice this recipe daily and be happy!

Hugs

The hug is a most valued tool for people. A baby could not develop without touch. It is the elderly that long for touch. Sometimes they are the forgotten ones. Whenever I visit someone I make sure I give them a hug—with their permission, of course. Rarely do I get "No" for an answer.

I'm 100 Today!

"I was nifty when I turned 50! Now, I'm 100 years old today!"

I asked, "How did you get to be 100?"

"I did it one day at a time—all by myself," she said with a huge grin and her hands on her hips!

"I see. Well, Happy Birthday and may God bless you with many more!

She smiled and said, "Thanks!"

An Elder's Life Instructions

I met with a group of residents at an independent living facility. I told them I wanted them to share with me their life instructions for a good life. They gave it a lot of thought before they responded, and I was surprised with their responses.

- Each day find someone you love and hug them. Let them know you care.
- Send a Valentine card to a friend or family member each year.
- Tell one joke daily and share a good laugh. (A clean joke that is!)
- Expect nothing great for your birthday and become happy with a big surprise.
- Smile instead of frown—it'll decrease those old-age wrinkles.
- Appreciate the simple things in your daily living.
- Accept the things you can't change and make the best of everything in your daily life.
- Whistle a happy tune in the shower.
- Marry only for love—even though you may think the money will make you happy for the moment.
- See the other person's point of view and try to not get too set in your ways.
- Make a new friend each month and let them know they're welcome to visit you at any time.
- Encourage a child to become successful and stay close to God with a strong faith.
- Celebrate your birthday each year with zest.
- Treat people kindly—like you would want to be treated.
- Love your neighbor as yourself.

- Be thoughtful of others.
- Read a Bible verse every day.
- Say a prayer of thanksgiving for each day you have left in your life.
- Pay someone a sincere complement—to either stranger or friend.
- Don't be afraid to admit a mistake because we are all human.
- Be humble upon your greatest accomplishment.
- Love yourself sincerely so you can shower your love on someone else.
- Help someone in need.
- Visit the sick or a shut in.
- Stay close to your family ties and children.
- Think before you speak.
- If you pick a fight, plan to fight your own fight.
- Be a good listener.
- Be a good sport.
- Always keep your promise.
- Never be a sore loser.
- If it isn't in black and white it didn't happen.
- Honor your mother and father until death you do part.
- When things happen—handle them.
- Take pride in whatever you do.
- Strive for excellence.
- Never cry over spilled milk.
- Too many hands in the broth, spoils the soup.
- If you don't use your head—you will use your feet.

Mary with Alzheimer's Disease
My Mother's Story

Mother liked to go out to eat, especially for lunch. She liked Reuben sandwiches. There is a little restaurant in Waukesha, Wisconsin, that makes the best Reubens. One time I picked Mother up on Valentine's Day at the care facility and I said, "How would you like to have a Reuben?"

"Fine," was Mother's answer.

We had our sandwich, and I made small talk to pass the time. She announced she needed to go to the bathroom. I started to go with her, but she was so independent that she fussed she could go alone. I watched and cringed as I saw her enter the Men's room. I ran after her to try to stop her. There was a man in there using the room. I spoke up immediately saying, "Mom! You are in the men's room. Sir, I am so sorry. Mother has Alzheimer's and did not read the sign." He whipped his head around and said, "Right lady!"

I learned to be gentle and assertive all in the same ball of wax! I always walked with her saying I, too, had to go to the bathroom and that kept the problem from happening again.

I continued to take Mom to lunch and for rides in the country because this was a pleasantry from her past that she so enjoyed.

Mary Before Alzheimer's

Mother and Father both grew up in Mishawaka, Indiana.

All through Mom's life she liked to ride in the country. She came to visit us in the summer and we always took her for a Sunday ride. She began trying to pronounce the names of the towns, such as Oconomowoc and Mukwonago. As she stumbled over the names she finally piped up and said, "Why don't they have easy names like Mishawaka?" At this point in the conversation my husband and I cracked a big smile.

Charity in the Love of My Mother

For many years I talked about doing charity work when I retired from catering. I was not sure what charity I would be affiliated with, but it became very clear to me when my mother was afflicted with Alzheimer's.

In May of 2000 I sold cookbooks at our parish to help raise money for the local Alzheimer's Association. I began to realize that I needed to enlarge my territory and to sell my books throughout the United States. I made a decision to donate my money, not only to the local Alzheimer's Association, but throughout the U.S. As I began my mission and traveled across the U.S., doing book signings and food classes at various libraries, I began to listen to people looking for help dealing with caring for an Alzheimer's loved one. I continued my work and answered questions and gave out information so these caregivers and their families could get help.

At my book signings I would serve milk and cookies. I patterned this after my mother's philosophy. When I was a little girl Mom would have milk and cookies for me when I arrived home from school. I would then tell her about my day. This same method of feeding people and listening to their stories has worked, and I am able to personally connect with people needing help.

When I was interviewed by the *Gwinnett Daily Post* they asked what I would say if I had one more chance to speak to my mother. My response was, "I love you and thank you. It was your burden with Alzheimer's that gave me the gift to reach out to the world and touch others. Your struggle turned into a blessing. One day, we'll whip up a whole bunch of potato salad for heaven. Just wait!"

I remembered when I was still at home I would make 100 pounds of potato salad each year on Dignus Day (a Polish holiday celebrated the day after Easter Sunday). Folks would get together at my parents' restaurant and dance. We served polish sausage and potato salad. I peeled all those potatoes and boiled and peeled the eggs. It was a big deal and a lot of work.

Aunt Gene

My Aunt Gene came to live in Wisconsin after my uncle died. She was afflicted with Alzheimer's, too. Her daughter, my cousin, and I grew close because we had a common bond. Aunt Gene was very docile while my mother was combative. Both of these women taught me so much about the disease and spurred me on to help others.

My Dad

He was witty and could be very charming. When I was a little girl he taught me how to swim and play volleyball. As I grew older he applauded me for doing well in college and showed he was very proud of me.

One day in October he called and asked if he could come and visit. I said, "Sure, Dad, you are welcome anytime."

When he arrived we ate and joked around as usual. He asked if we could go for a ride in the country. As we were riding he announced his time on this earth was short. "I just wanted to come and reassure you that you have been a good daughter and I love you very much." Three months later he passed away with colon cancer. This was a hard visit, but a good one. Our times together meant so much to me.

Life is a Journey
by Pat Nekola

Life is a journey with peaks and valleys.
Sweetened with the good smells of the
Lily of the Valley.

Life is what you make of it.
God dealt each person a hand of cards.
He is relying on you to play your cards right.
So journey with your hand of cards to the fullest of your ability.

Journey through life using your head, hands, and heart.
Inspire and nurture a child
And take care of one elder person in your life
To make this world a better place to live.

To have lived at least once you must
Journey to the beach, dig your toes in the sand,
And feel the rays of sun on your face.
To have loved someone and have someone love you.

When you are on a journey, caring for an elder parent,
Take time for yourself and reflect,
Knowing you have made this a better place
By giving your loving care to your parent,
Your reward is great in the kingdom of heaven.

A Beautiful Story for a Beautiful Woman of Faith

by Elizabeth Wessa

Sister Dolores Pertzborn, known in her younger days as Sister Theorita, has given 60 years of her life to the community and religious life. She states she has oodles of memories!

She was born in Springfield Corners, Wisconsin, on a small farm, the ninth child in a family of twelve. Her family consisted of six boys and six girls. She had loving parents. The children helped do the chores, but they also had fun playing baseball.

One time she was driving the horses on a hay wagon. "As we climbed one of the many hilly areas on our farm, the haystack was piling up. I fell off the front of the wagon and landed in between the two horses. They stood perfectly still until Pa could rescue me. . . . Even though there were twelve of us, Pa would take us one-by-one to town and buy a five-cent ice cream cone. He loved ice cream and our whole family did, too. I enjoyed coming from a family of twelve!"

Sister Dolores attended school in a three-room school at St. Martin in Martinsville, Wisconsin. She did not know any English when she started first grade, as the family spoke German. Sister Dolores lost a brother at age five from leukemia and another brother at age 18. He was killed instantly in a car accident on Memorial Day weekend.

She and her family experienced grief and it was their faith that carried them through.

When she was thinking about becoming a Sister she decided to talk to her pa about it.

His response was, "When God wanted my son He didn't ask me. If God wants you to be a Sister and you want to be a Sister, you may go with my blessing."

She joined the convent in 1940, and has spent a lifetime serving others with faith and love. Her good example has touched my life.

One of the students from a Psychology class asked Sister Dolores if she would want to be a teenager these days. Her answer was, "No, I wouldn't want to be a teenager again. I am happy with the experiences I had. I do enjoy seeing youngsters and watching their vibrancy, but teenagers have so many more challenges now than when I was a teen."

Then the student asked: "Do you feel society sends a message to people your age?"

"Yes, even though I am old, there are still things I can learn and accomplish. A number of years ago society viewed anyone over 60 as fit only for retirement, but now society thinks nothing of someone my age still working. Society is more open in that sense. Someone won't necessarily hire another person based on their agc, rathcr they hire people with the abilities to do the job well."

"What is negative about being your age, Sister?"

"Something that is negative about being my age is not being able to do all the things I would like to do. For example, I can't stay up late anymore because I get too tired. I also know that my sense of hearing isn't what it used to be. Luckily my eyesight is still good. I rarely need to wear my glasses. I don't appreciate people who say they are younger than they really are. They pretend they can still do the same things they used to do. This is not true, you can't do all the things you want, but you need to accept that you are growing older."

"What are your favorite memories from your youth?"

"I really remember playing baseball with my family. That was a lot of fun. I remember loving school and visiting relatives a lot. That's somewhat of a lost art now. Back then, we knew all of our cousins and we would visit them and get to know them better. I also remember helping make hay on the farm. I enjoyed that a lot. That was a job that helped mark you as growing up."

"Do you feel your life has been fulfilling?"

"Yes, I feel my life has been very fulfilling. I have had a variety of opportunities and I do not feel that I have missed out on anything in my life. I have traveled to Europe and have had so many opportunities to do things. I have enjoyed them because I feel they have made my life very rich."

Sister Dolores is a wonderful, vibrant person. She is extremely friendly and accommodating. She is insightful and very interesting. She is a real role model. I hope when I reach my later seventies I will be as vibrant. Sister Dolores continues her ministry with children. "Children have played a vital role in becoming the person I am," said Sister Dolores. For the past sixty years she has touched many people. I honor her for her service and dedication.

Good Advice

While making my rounds I spoke with a gentleman named Glen as he reflected on his life. He said, "Life is God's most precious gift. Live it to the fullest!"

"Let kindness to the elderly make many pictures in the scrapbook of reflections."—Pat Nekola.

A Friend's Grandmother

I first met my friend's grandmother at my friend's engagement party. Her grandmother was a very sharp lady and the life of the party. She was so happy for my friend to be marrying such a nice, young man. She was also very proud of her granddaughter.

Her grandmother was a colorful person. She liked to play cards with her grandchildren and participate in family outings and reunions. She wasn't afraid to speak her mind, either. She enjoyed the latest fashions and styles and was a very sharp dresser—even at 90 years of age. She had a hat for every occasion.

She always claimed that if you participate in life and be with the young people, you, yourself, will stay young.

On the day of her funeral family members and friends wore a hat in honor of their Grandmother!

The Red Hat Club

While traveling through Illinois I stopped at one of the local libraries in East Central Illinois. As I entered the library a meeting was going on with ladies wearing red hats. There were all kinds and styles of red hats. Most of the ladies were senior citizens.

One lady was a "stitch"! She was wearing an outfit with nothing that matched. She stated that she's old enough that she will wear what she pleases and not take any more orders!

I told her, "I'm with you sweetheart! I hate polyester pants. If any caregiver ever puts plaid polyester pants with a striped polyester top on me, I'm going to give her a lamb chop!"

"That a girl!" the red hat lady exclaimed.

The club ladies were trying to solve the world's problems and having a grand time together.

I have since learned that the Red Hat Club exists all over the U.S. The babysitter I had while growing up belongs to a Red Hat Club in Indiana.

Thoughts About Time,
from Adele

Time has passed so quickly.
In my younger years I worried so about small things.
They don't mean much to me anymore.
Why does one have to grow old to gain the wisdom of
Understanding the true meaning of time?

I no longer dust because the dust has a way of finding
Its way back to the same spot again.
I'm glad I don't see the dust—for it does not matter
To me anymore.

When I get a visitor rapping on my door,
I just say, "Come in.
Thank you for checking on me today and thank you for
The pretty lilacs from your garden. It was so sweet that
You took time to visit me today.
I will worry no more about tomorrow, but enjoy today."

Thank you, Lord, for one more day.
For today I will take time as I reflect on the good
Memories in my life.

My Pig Story

While traveling through the Midwest I was scheduled to give a picnic program for caregivers. They were caring for Alzheimer's parents or family members. It was a night out for them.

Respite care is very vital to be a good caregiver. I can't stress that enough!

A gentleman from the Alzheimer's Association was present to introduce me and he also spoke about Alzheimer's Disease and the importance of education when becoming a caregiver.

While preparing the food one person asked me why I had a big pig sitting up on the demonstration table. "Well," I said, "if you make breakfast a chicken gives a contribution of eggs. But the pig gives the bacon and makes a real commitment. I am committed to a mission in honor of my mom to help raise funds to educate caregivers to improve the quality of life for the Alzheimer's patients and also to help caregivers keep their sanity."

At that point a lady raised her hand and stood up. She was wearing a beautiful hat with a rainbow of colors. The brim of the hat was turned up as the colors continued the rainbow effect. She took her hat off and said, "Your pig needs a hat. I lost my mom to Alzheimer's. This was her favorite hat. She always wore it to her card club, for good luck."

"I can't take it," I said. "It has sentimental value to you."

"No, please take this hat for good luck. Your pig really needs a hat as you travel in honor of my mom, too."

I asked her to come to the front and place the hat on the pig's head, and I threw my arms around her and hugged her. I thanked her for the wonderful gesture and vowed that the pig would wear the hat everywhere I gave picnic talks. To this day I continue to carry my pig with the hat and I relate this heartfelt hat story.

She Calls Me "Mama"

At one of the facilities where I play my accordion, Sara always greets me upon arrival with a, "Hi Mama!"

She holds her baby doll and sings every word of the old-time songs. Her face is illuminated with much joy, and it is such a pleasure to play for her.

She Calls Me by Name

At the same facility another lady always calls me by my name. I ask myself how can this be? She has Alzheimer's. She also helps me distribute and collect the rhythmic instruments. She always says, "See you next time."

Her Alzheimer's condition has progressed slowly so she can still enjoy the little pleasantries in life. She is a sweet person.

One of My Favorite Places

For three years I traveled to a certain care facility. It was an older facility, but the people were cared for and loved very deeply. The cost to take good care of the people continued to soar and they asked for donations and did fundraising to help keep the facility open. With the sinking economic problems they finally had to close. My heart ached when this announcement came to me. I loved the people there and enjoyed doing activities with them.

I receive many thank you notes and letters of praise, but this letter was so special it made me teary-eyed. This special letter helps spur me on in my work.

Dear Staff,

A good nursing home is many things. It's a place of healing, security, nurturing, and care. It's a place of friendship, laughter, music, and joy. It's a place where quality of life is a constant goal and a deep commitment. But all of this cannot change the fact that a nursing home, like the work in general, is also, at times—a place of pain and suffering, loneliness, and loss.

What makes the healing laughter possible? What makes the suffering and loss bearable? It is shared love, compassion, and companionship.

The contributions you have made to our facility, dear friend, have spoken loudly of love and have become part of the glue that has held this tired, old place together for so many years. We hope you are able to remember and to feel blessed by the look in the eye of this or that resident who responded gratefully to the gift of your presence. We hope you have a sense of significance of those smiles that appeared as our goodness moved and touched their hearts. We pray you feel a wholeness that comes from sharing of one's self with God's people in need.

We, who have worked at this facility, will always hold a special place for you in our memories and in our hearts. You have added texture and spice to lives that deserved the best we could give them.

May God bless you and keep you; and until we meet again, may he hold you in the palm of His hand.

Thank you.

So as the doors closed on one of my favorite facilities I said my goodbyes to all the beautiful people I came to love.

I began to reflect on some of the memories I made at that facility.

Jimmy was still wanting to go fishing on a big boat. He continued to tell me the big fish stories of the one that got away. These stories brought him great pleasure.

Peaches was fussing over her stuffed animals and fun gadget gifts from her family. She was quite a lady and loved teatime.

I remember celebrating *Kate's* 100th birthday and her having great fun at her party.

There was *Lee* singing every song, word-for-word and enjoying my accordion music.

Chris was still planning family parties and wanting to go shopping soon.

Sara told her stories about working in Africa.

Theresa always wanted to hold my hand.

Elizabeth called out to her husband, begging him to take her home.

Marge was still rocking her baby, for she was a mother of seven and still playing her motherly role, even at the age of 90.

Harry was still asking me to play the song "Good Night Irene" as he proclaimed he should have never let Irene go away.

This experience has created fond memories for me and has touched my life forever.

Abuse

I stopped at a library to speak on Alzheimer's. A lady in the group seemed depressed and I asked her if she was all right.

She told me she was caring for her mother-in-law, who had Alzheimer's. She was up most of the night with her mother-in-law.

When I talked with her she began to cry and said "I lost my patience with her and was verbally abusive, and I feel so bad."

I said anyone can lose their patience. What could you have done to avoid this—or even better what can you do so this doesn't occur again? After rehearsing with her she realized she needed to change her ideas and go with the flow. I wished her well as I left.

I think of her and hope she is managing all right. She did make it very clear she did not want to abuse her mother-in-law. She was just getting very frustrated and is very sad for her mother-in-law.

Harmony

As caregivers we need to have patience and be compassionate. I think of it as being a weaver with vibrant colors of threads that all mess together in a wholesome way. A caregiver must be strong and healthy. Throughout your day you must be a juggler, moving from one situation to another.

Because the afflicted come from all walks of life and are thrown into a melting pot of personalities and situations they must learn to live side-by-side in harmony at their facility. (Kind of like weaving those threads into a beautiful fabric.) With encouragement each person can nourish and enrich the beauty of the others.

We ask the Master Weaver for patience, compassion, and peace. Remember there are many facets of caregiving.

When I worked full time at a local facility I promoted the premise that we were a family and we needed to be considerate of each other. For the most part I found people willing to try my approach and be considerate of everyone.

Words of Wisdom from the Elderly

People are People.

They say you can't judge a book by its cover.

People come in all shapes and sizes with all different personalities and from different walks of life.

Each person has talents and abilities to enrich this earth.

People can make others happy, sad, or blue. People can love or hate. But whatever you do—think before you act.

The multi-colors of butterflies fly high against the sky for young and old alike to enjoy—for beauty is in the eyes of the beholder.

The wonder of nature and beauty go hand-in-hand.

The world is lovely with the sounds of the birds.

The fragrant smells of spring flowers make a person feel so young.

Food for Thought,
Advice from the Elderly

This is a beautiful world when people are kind and considerate of each other. It is people helping people that make the difference.

You will reap what you sow.

The wonders of nature tell me there is a God.

Beauty is in the eyes of the beholder.

Act enthusiastic and be enthusiastic!

Work a full day for a fair day's wages.

A friend in need, is a friend indeed.

Be a ham and laugh a lot.

Take gossip with a grain of salt.

When you can't sleep just count your blessings!

Say a prayer for America.

Show your support for your family and friends.

Help a stranger.

Think big!

Enjoy each day of your life.

Stay active and healthy.

Put your trust in the Lord and He will carry you a lifetime.

Live your life one day at a time.

If a person harms you once—shame on them, but if you let them harm you twice—shame on you.

Forgive and forget.

Live by the book of the golden rule.

The world is a better place because of knowledge and technology.

Different strokes for different folks makes the world more interesting.

The world is beautiful when people make the difference for each other.

Traveling in South Carolina

While traveling in South Carolina I met a young man who was very committed to serving the elderly. He gained interest in this by watching his parents care for his grandmother. He felt the need to follow this path in life and his professor encouraged him to study Gerontology.

After he graduated he began working with the elderly and eventually he took a position with the Alzheimer's Association. They were developing an art program in California and Colorado and he wanted to follow the same program in his home area.

He said, "There is nothing wrong with Bingo or watching TV, but something more is needed to stimulate this group of people." He wanted to provide a more structured art activity that was 'failure free' (no right or wrong outcome), and designed specifically for the Alzheimer's residents.

He contacted the state arts commission and said, "You have wonderful art projects for the young, but there is nothing for the elderly. I would like you to help the elderly with some art programs."

The commission reviewed his ideas and suggestions and they were able to supply a grant for this valuable program called "Caring Colors". This program continues to be funded each year, even though there have been state budget cuts.

Two Success Stories

There was a lady who declined participating in any activities, but she got involved in the "Caring Colors" program. She produced beautiful art and maintained her attention span to make beautiful memories.

There was also a very withdrawn gentleman at this same facility. He got involved in the "Caring Colors" program and the man began talking again. It changed his disposition greatly.

Everyone needs a purpose in life!

She Misses Him

A couple of years ago I met a young man named Chris and his wife, Rhonda Callahan. They are a beautiful couple, both having studied social work. Chris is working with Alzheimer's patients singing his music and playing his guitar.

This song was sung by Chris at a caregiver's breakfast. There was not a dry-eyed person in the group. The singer said he had a hard time not crying, too. The lyrics about say it all—you lose your loved one twice.

She shaves his face.
She combs his hair.
She helps him find his rocking chair.
She cooks his meals.
She wipes his mouth—and the window that he is looking out.
She reads him books.
She speaks his name.
Oh, every day is much the same.
She sighs that sigh from deep within,
She's one that says she misses him.
She misses his gentle touch and the way he used to make her laugh.
She misses the man he was in all those old photographs.
So strong, so kind, so sweet, so smart,
The man who stole her very heart.
She misses him.
His children come on Saturday.
They are at his feet,
His grandkids play.
It is sad that they don't know him at all.
He's just the one they call, Grandpa.
They take out his trash.
They mow the lawn.
Things he can't do since he's been gone.

She's grateful they are pitching in,
And like everyone, she misses him.
Yes, they're still together after all these years,
But sometime you can almost feel the sadness in her tears.

Chris has made a CD called "Memories". There are four songs on the disk. These songs are dedicated to caregivers that carry the memories of those who no longer can. The songs will touch your heart forever.

1. *"She Misses Him", written by Tim Johnson, EMI Blackwood Music, Inc. Background music by Stellar Records, Inc.*
2. *"You've Got a Friend", written by Carole King, Colgems-EMI Music Inc. Background music by Sound Choice.*
3. *"Somebody's Praying", written by John G. Elliot, BMG Songs, Inc. Acoustic Guitar by Chris Callahan. Percussion by Chris Callahan and bass guitar by Doug Fulton.*
4. *"Memories", written by Chris and Rhonda Callahan. Acoustic guitar by Chris Callahan. Percussion by Chris Callahan and bass guitar by Doug Fulton.*

All proceeds benefit the Alzheimer's Association in the Canton Area Chapter. There are many more dedicated people working for the Alzheimer's Association to help families—and their kind efforts show!

A Father and Son Story

Fathers want their sons to excel and succeed in life.

From little on up, Dad and son ran races together. They ran the same marathon every year. At the age of 55, the father ran with his 19-year-old son.

The father was always there encouraging his son to run—and to win.

On the day of the marathon they started the race together. At first the father kept up, but eventually he fell back in the pack of racers. His son won the race! The father was so proud of his son and congratulated him on his victory.

One year later the father's mental health was failing, and he was diagnosed with Alzheimer's Disease. The son visited him often. However, as the disease progressed it became harder to visit his father, and the older man didn't recognize his son.

On one visit the son mentioned how they ran those races together and his father replied, "And wasn't it great how I kept up with you and even outran you?" Even though the father was in his own little world, a memory was triggered for a moment!

My Husband's Question

My husband asked me, "What are you going to do if you end up having to care for me with Alzheimer's? Will you feel cheated or angry?"

I said, "I'll feel sad, but you can count on me to be there with you, and for you, every step of the way."

"Thank you," he said.

Ice Cream

John liked his ice cream! He said the world would be a better place if everyone could eat one extra scoop of ice cream with someone special every day. Then there would a whole lot of less-lonely people.

A Treasured Trunk Brings Back Old Memories

One day Mary Agnes dug through her grandma's trunk only to find a host of memories.

There were pictures of her grandma and grandpa's wedding day. They were such a handsome couple! Grandpa always wore a full mustache and Grandma had big eyes. (Maybe that is why she could see if there was any trouble.)

Mary Agnes didn't remember ever seeing her grandpa wear a suit. "Do you suppose his wedding day was the only day he dressed up for Grandma?" she asked herself. Grandma's wedding dress had puff sleeves and dainty lace trim and she wore a broad-brimmed hat trimmed with flowers. "Grandma always wore hats," Mary Agnes thought to herself, remembering Grandma's beautiful pearl hatpin.

Grandma came from Belgium when she was in her later teen years and Grandpa was from Holland. Grandma told of being almost shipwrecked on her voyage and she never went near water for the rest of her life.

Grandpa loved to tell this story about Grandma. He boasted how he had fooled Grandma about his age because she had said she never wanted to marry an older man.

It was love at first sight when they met. Grandpa never told her his correct age, but said he was two years older than she was because he was afraid she wouldn't marry him if she *knew* he was really twelve years older! So, Grandpa lied about his age. They had been married ten years and had six children before Grandma found out the truth! She was a little upset, but Grandpa said, "Sorry Ma, it's a little too late to change your mind now."

There was an antique tablecloth in the trunk. Grandma had used it for her formal holiday dinners. Mary Agnes held it up to her face and hugged it as she thought about how she loved to go to Grandma's house for holiday fun. She remembered Grandma making the fresh, homemade bread, churned butter, and the great homemade pies, too.

At those family gatherings Grandpa always said they had plenty to eat during the Depression days because he planted a variety of fruit trees and a huge vegetable garden. They also raised chickens and so they always had the basics and good home-baked desserts. Grandma's homemade strawberry rhubarb pie was the best!

Uncle Herman attended every holiday event, as he was a bachelor. He loved desserts. He always said you should eat your dessert first, then the meat and potatoes. He always liked to sit next to Mary Agnes as she always gave him her piece of pie. Uncle Herman always said she was his favorite niece, but she wondered if it was really so, or if he just wanted her dessert.

Aunt Sophie liked to play with the children at the family gatherings. She would put one hand on each cheek and move the child's head back and forth until they were dizzy. Sophie was a big tease. One day when they were playing tag Sophie fell and broke her wrist. That was the last game of tag!

Grandpa always said Aunt Bet should be taught to listen (she was such a talker), and she might become a little wiser!

Uncle Benny was a little rough around the edges—but

he had a kind heart. He would sing "Reuben, Reuben, I've been thinking, what the heck have you been drinking? Is it beer or is it wine—heck no! It's turpentine!" By the time the song was finished all the children would be giggling.

Mary Agnes remembered Grandma's hexagon poker tabletop. Grandma got a little too enthusiastic about playing poker sometimes.

After dinner was all cleaned up and the dishes and food put away, the adults would play poker for pennies.

Grandma had a set of neat black and red shiny poker chips.

The kids would all go outside to play ball or roll in the snow while the adults were playing poker. Mary Agnes always seemed to look rumpled after their games and her mother always told her she would win the prize for being untidy.

Mary Agnes sighed as she closed the trunk and left more memories for another day—those were the good old days!

Friends and Family

My mother-in-law always said, "You pick your friends, but not your family. So stay close to your friends all your life."

She always enjoyed shopping, visiting, and playing bridge with her friends.

My in-laws moved into an apartment complex as my father-in-law's health began to fail. He was mentally sharp until his death. He loved to watch the school kids play ball at recess. He made it clear to me throughout my life that it is the little things in life that count. So enjoy!

My Purpose

Everyone needs a purpose in life.

I am very blessed to have had the opportunity to work with the elderly, for their wisdom has touched my heart forever.

I am thanking my mother, again, for without her Alzheimer's condition I would have never experienced this chapter of my life. I know that my God and Lord gives me my invisible hug in my daily living. I have truly reaped the benefits.

An Alzheimer's Story

I have Alzheimer's. You need to know more than what you see about me. If I could only remember and express myself, I would try to tell you in my own words about my thoughts—the best I know how.

Here it goes . . .

I may be growing older and my memory going a little slower. My feet don't often go where I want them to go—instead they shuffle along.

Please don't speak to me in such a demeaning way. I have very deep feelings, lost in this body of mine. Sometimes the words just don't come out right. I may be getting slower, but I am not dead.

My eyes can't see what you think I should see. I'm in my own little world and you need to accept what I can see. Please understand that as my disease progresses my memory will continue to diminish, but my feelings will always be intact.

My hearing has diminished, but I can hear what you say about me, and to me, when I want to hear it! I have learned "selective hearing". Don't you see? I do listen, but sometimes I pretend your words are missing. Then I can cope better—for I no longer understand your world, or can participate with you on your terms.

The emotional ties are slowly going downhill as I continue to slip away, against my will, to the twilight zone.

You will lose me twice, my love, once to Alzheimer's and then to death—one inch at a time. But I am *still* here in body and spirit, even though my mind is slowly leaving me.

I can still enjoy the pretty colors of flowers and the fragrant smells of nature. I can still enjoy parts of my day. I still like to see the squirrels scurry up the tree and I love the breeze on my blank face.

I still like to have someone hold my hand and walk with me in the park. I like to stir up a big batch of chocolate chip cookies. I love the smell of bread baking—I just don't remember all the steps and need a little help.

I get tired of faking trying to fit into your world. But my mind just will not permit me to do what you want me to do any longer.

I want to be a part of your daily activities, and be important—even though my attention span has shortened. I have been assigned a new journey in life as I go down this crooked path.

I am sorry if I'm a burden—or cause you pain. Please understand I can't remember your name any longer, for I am not the same.

Dear Lord,

Make every person in my daily life love and respect me and also treat me with dignity for being a new person.

Hold my hand sweet Jesus, as I journey down this crooked road with Alzheimer's.

Lord, I am in your hands and I'm counting on you for your kind support.

Thank you, sweet Jesus.

—Amen

Caregiver's Responses

I took my dad to the doctor today. The doctor said Dad has the start of Alzheimer's Disease.

I denied it. I went home and screamed and pounded my fist on the table, "No! He *does not* have Alzheimer's. He is just a little forgetful. Anyone could forget to turn off the stove, or run a red light. My dad will be just fine as long as he stays in his home."

I don't want to lose you Mom. I love you so much. It is my fault that I didn't come more often to see you and only telephoned you. I'll make it up to you. I am going to care for you every step of the way. I'm here for you.

Why do I have to continue to repeat these directions so often? Why can't he/she remember just a little something? I'm trying to give clues.

A caregiver begs her brother to come to see their dad. He responds, "Please don't ask me to come to see Dad. I live 2,000 miles away. I just want to remember him the way he was when we went fishing and when we had good times together. I don't want to know what Alzheimer's is all about, I may just be in his shoes one day. What I don't know won't hurt me."

Some of Pat's Experiences

For the most part the majority of caregivers I've encountered want to do their very best for their loved one.

There is so much to learn to do a good job. A caregiver needs to take care of herself/himself before they can take care of someone else. They need to keep this in mind, as taking care of an Alzheimer's patient is a 24-7 job.

I Think I Remember What I Wanted to Eat

A couple was still living in their home even though they both had Alzheimer's Disease.

One day when they returned from their doctor appointments they decided they had a taste for ice cream.

The husband said, "You relax, I'll get the ice cream. By the way, what would you like on your ice cream?"

"I'd like chocolate and whipped cream with a cherry on top."

He proceeded to the kitchen and prepared a large ham sandwich for the two of them to share. When he returned he was all smiles.

"Honey, here is your sandwich."

She replied, "Gil you forgot the mustard for the sandwich."

Jamie and Jeannie

Jeannie had her daughter, Jamie, out of wedlock when she was 17. Jeannie never married. She struggled to raise her daughter and there was always a great deal of tension between the two of them. Jeannie constantly worried about Jamie repeating her mother's mistakes. Jeannie's parents tried to be supportive and they were good grandparents to Jamie.

Jamie lacked self-confidence, and her mother seemed to nag constantly about one thing or another. There was a power struggle between these two women. Jamie would scream at her mother and say, "I hate you. When I grow up I'm leaving for good and never coming back!" When she was grown she moved to New York City and became a model. Due to the family friction she didn't go home very much.

It was her day off and Jamie was at home relaxing when the telephone rang.

"Hi Jamie, this is your mother. I just came from the doctor and there is something I need to tell you. I have been diagnosed with Alzheimer's Disease. I want to tell you now before I get worse that I have always loved you. I suppose I was not only fearful, but also jealous of you. Please forgive me, Jamie. Can you please come home and see me before it is too late and I can no longer communicate?"

Jamie hung up the phone and sobbed. She was speechless, and her heart ached. She spent the next week considering options for her mother's care and made the decision to go home and care for her mother through her journey with Alzheimer's.

Jamie spent one year with her mother. In that year she thanked God for this great opportunity to finally become a loving family. She asked her mom for forgiveness for saying she hated her. The Alzheimer's Disease became a blessing for them.

Other Alzheimer's Stories

There was a grumpy, old man at one of the facilities I visited. We tried to get him involved in activities thinking it would help his disposition, but he refused.

One day one of the staff members got the idea that it would be good for him to have a job, so we asked him if he would like the job of feeding the fish.

He was very possessive of *his* fish! They were his fish and he would take care of them! We went right along with him in this regard. His job improved his disposition immensely!

At another facility the nurse didn't believe in letting the women patients hold or rock dolls.

We had a patient there with sun-downing problems. One day when the nurse was not there we got a doll for Marian to rock and cuddle. It seemed to quiet her down. Then Marion proceeded to pick up her top and loosen her bra—preparing to breast feed her baby. Unfortunately, the nurse returned, so we rushed Marion into her room and let her feed her baby in her own little world.

"Please Take Me Home"

"I want to go home!" Myrtle said.

"You are at home," Missy replied.

"No, I am not! I want to go home!"

Missy asked, "Mom, where is home?"

Myrtle was back in her childhood days and she told about her home on the farm where she grew up.

Remember, Alzheimer's patients go back to their childhood days. Their short-term memory is lost—but their long-term memory stays intact for a much longer time.

A person can live as long as 20 years with Alzheimer's. The average length is eight years.

Half of the elder population has some form of dementia after the age of 85. Alzheimer's can strip a person's mind and turn them into a vegetable as the person returns to the fetal position in the end stage of the disease.

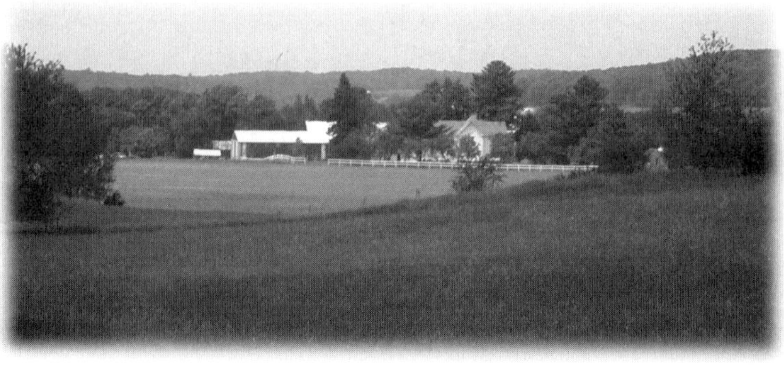

Information included in Part One of this Handbook:

- *Easy to understand information on each stage of the disease.*
- *How to deal with the different stages for families and caregivers.*
- *Coping strategies when caring for the patient at home.*
- *What to look for when selecting a care facility.*
- *Resources including telephone numbers, websites, and questions to ask.*

Information and Activities Useful for the Care Facilities' Activity Directors included in Part Two of this Handbook:

- *Directions for different craft activities.*
- *Color graphics for use with the activities.*
- *Recommended music for patient participation.*
- *Recipes.*
- *Patient assessment forms.*

An Alzheimer's Guide

Activities and Issues for People Who Care

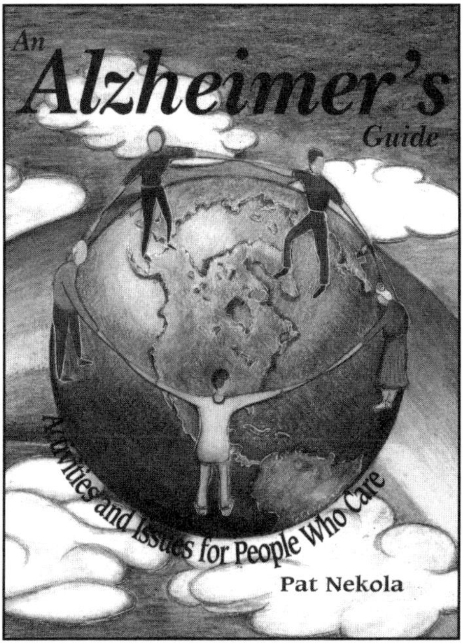

212 pages, soft cover.

ISBN: 0-9660610-9-8

Mail or fax to:
Catering by Design
P.O. Box 181
Waukesha, WI 53187
Ph: (262) 547-2004
Fax: (262) 547-8594

Customer Name ______________________________

Library ______________________________

Address ______________________________

City State Zip ______________________________

Phone ______________ Fax ______________

Qty:	Price @	Ext.
	$34.95	$
Shipping	$4.50	$
Total		$

MasterCard and Visa accepted.

WI residents please add 5.5% sales tax.

Signature ______________________________

Date ______________________________

Invoice Number ______________________________

Pat Nekola was born in Akron, Ohio, and raised in Indiana. She holds B.S. and M.A. degrees in home economics education with a minor in music. Pat became interested in helping the elderly when her mother became afflicted with Alzheimer's. She completed the ACT (Activity Consultant Trainers) and Management program sponsored by the state of Wisconsin and has worked as an Activity Director.

She presently travels the country conducting seminars with Activity staff in care facilities; counsels families dealing with Alzheimer's; and trains Girl Scouts to entertain the residents in local care facilities. She presents programs in libraries on Alzheimer's and picnics having written two previous books, *An Alzheimer's Guide—Activities and Issues for People Who Care*, and *Picnics—Catering on the Move: A Cookbook and Guide*.

Pat has been a co-facilitator for the Alzheimer's patients and gives a portion of her book sales to the Alzheimer's Association in honor of her mother. She is a strong advocate for the elderly, and has designed many activity programs for the elderly. Pat uses her programs to work with the elderly on a personal level.

Elder Activities *for People Who Care*

Volume One

January through June

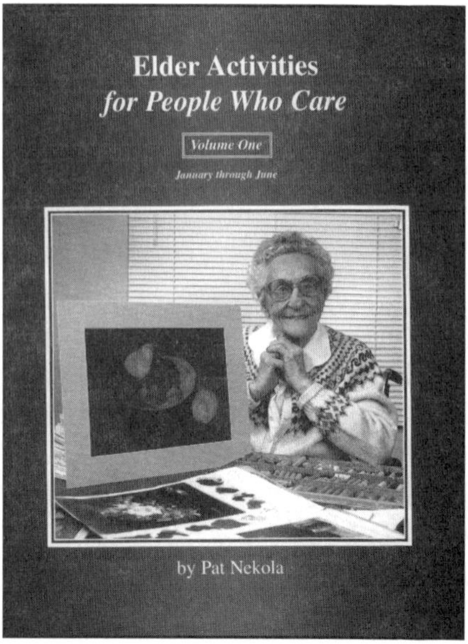

292 pages, soft cover.

ISBN: 0-9660610-8-X

Mail or fax to: Catering by Design
P.O. Box 181 • Waukesha, WI 53187
Ph: (262) 547-2004 • Fax: (262) 547-8594

Customer Name ______________________________

Library ______________________________

Address ______________________________

City State Zip ______________________________

Phone ____________________ Fax ____________________

Qty:	Price @	Ext.
	$34.95	$
Shipping	$4.50	$
Total		$

MasterCard and Visa accepted.

WI residents please add 5.5% sales tax.

Signature ______________________________

Date ______________________________

Invoice Number ______________________________

COMING SOON

Pat Nekola was born in Akron, Ohio, and raised in Indiana. She holds B.S. and M.A. degrees in home economics education with a minor in music. Pat became interested in helping the elderly when her mother became afflicted with Alzheimer's. She completed the ACT (Activity Consultant Trainers) and Management program sponsored by the state of Wisconsin and has worked as an Activity Director.

She presently travels the country conducting seminars with Activity staff in care facilities; counsels families dealing with Alzheimer's; and trains Girl Scouts to entertain the residents in local care facilities. She presents programs in libraries on Alzheimer's and picnics having written two previous books, *An Alzheimer's Guide—Activities and Issues for People Who Care*, and *Picnics—Catering on the Move: A Cookbook and Guide*.

Pat has been a co-facilitator for the Alzheimer's patients and gives a portion of her book sales to the Alzheimer's Association in hon... of her mother. She is a strong advocate for the elderly, and has designed many activity prog... for the elderly. Pat uses her programs to work with th... elderly on a personal level.

Elder Activities *for People Who Care*

Volume Two
July through December

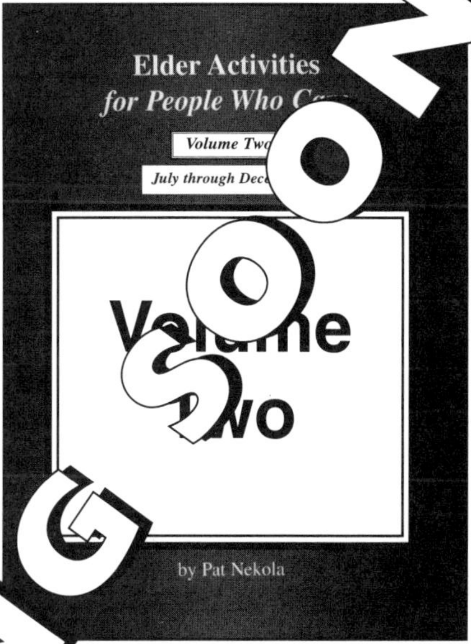

? pages, soft cover.

ISBN: 0-0000000-0-X

Mail ... ax to: Catering by Design
...Box 181 • Waukesha, WI 53187
...) 547-2004 • Fax: (262) 547-8594

Customer Name ______________________

Library ______________________

Address ______________________

City Sta ______________________

Ph ______________ Fax ______________

	Price @	Ext.
	$34.95	$
Shipping	$4.50	$
Total		$

MasterCard and Visa accepted.

WI residents please add 5.5% sales tax.

Signature ______________________

Date ______________________

Invoice Number ______________________